Let's Talk About Masks

A Children's Book and Conversation Starter for Parents

by Sara Jo Walker

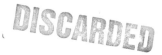

emerge
publishing

25 24 23 22 21 20   9 8 7 6 5 4 3 2 1

LET'S TALK ABOUT MASKS–A CHILDREN'S BOOK AND CONVERSATION STARTER FOR PARENTS

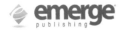

Published by:
Emerge Publishing, LLC
9521 Riverside Parkway, Suite 243 Tulsa, OK 74137
Phone: 888.407.4447 www.EmergePublishing.com

Library of Congress Cataloging-in-Publication Data:
ISBN: 978-1-949758-73-3 Paperback

BISAC:
JNF024020 JUVENILE NONFICTION/ Diseases, Illnesses & Injuries
JNF024080 JUVENILE NONFICTION / Health & Daily Living / Safety
JNF024000 JUVENILE NONFICTION / Health & Daily Living / General

Author Image by Laura Purtee Productions

Image credits:

wavebreakmedia/shutterstock.com
In Green/shutterstock.com
Sergey Mironov/shutterstock.com
Andrii Spy_k/shutterstock.com
Vladi333/shutterstock.com
Dmytro Zinkevych/shutterstock.com
Roman Samborskyi/shutterstock.com
Djile/shutterstock.com
Marcus Bay/shutterstock.com
FamVeld/shutterstock.com
VGstockstudio/shutterstock.com
Syda Productions/shutterstock.com
Inna Reznik/shutterstock.com
KatarinaTati/shutterstock.com
TY Lim/shutterstock.com
Explorich/shutterstock.com
Mix and Match Studio/shutterstock.com
sirtravelalot/shutterstock.com
Bell Ka Pang/shutterstock.com

Dedication

For Jack and Ivy.

You are my world!

Why do people wear masks?

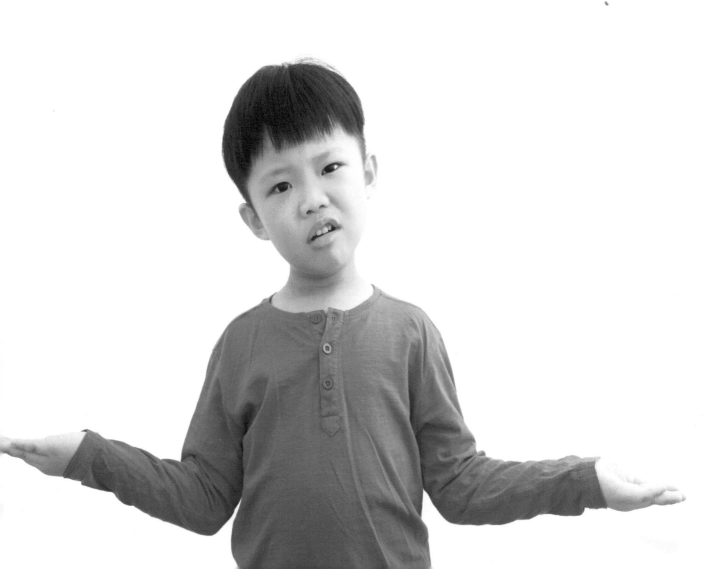

People all over the world wear
masks for many different reasons.

Most of the time, people wear masks
to protect themselves from getting hurt
or sick, or to keep from spreading germs.

Let's take a look at some people
that wear masks and find out why?

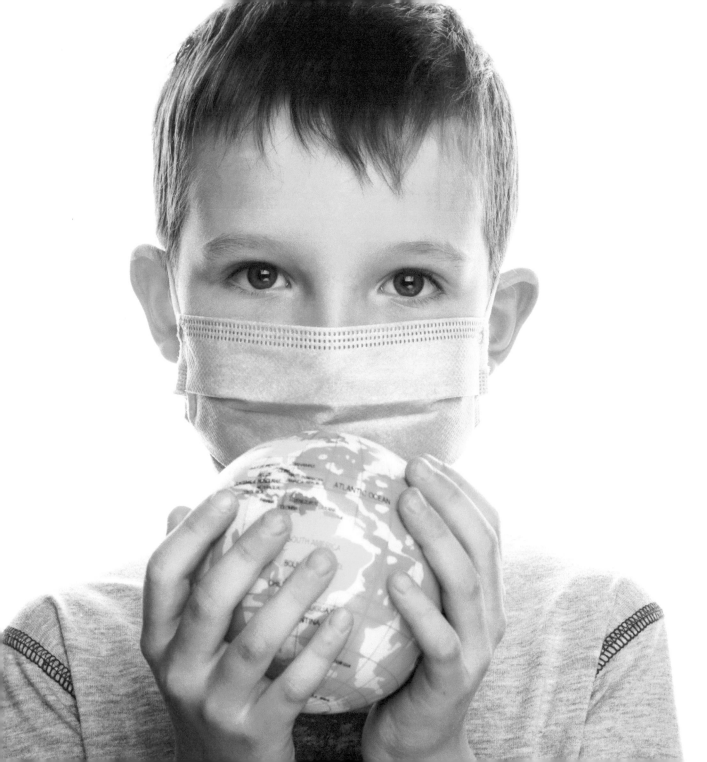

Fire Fighters Wear Masks

Fire fighters wear masks to keep from breathing in smoke and bad gasses caused by fires.

Masks help keep fire fighters safe so they can help other people to safety.

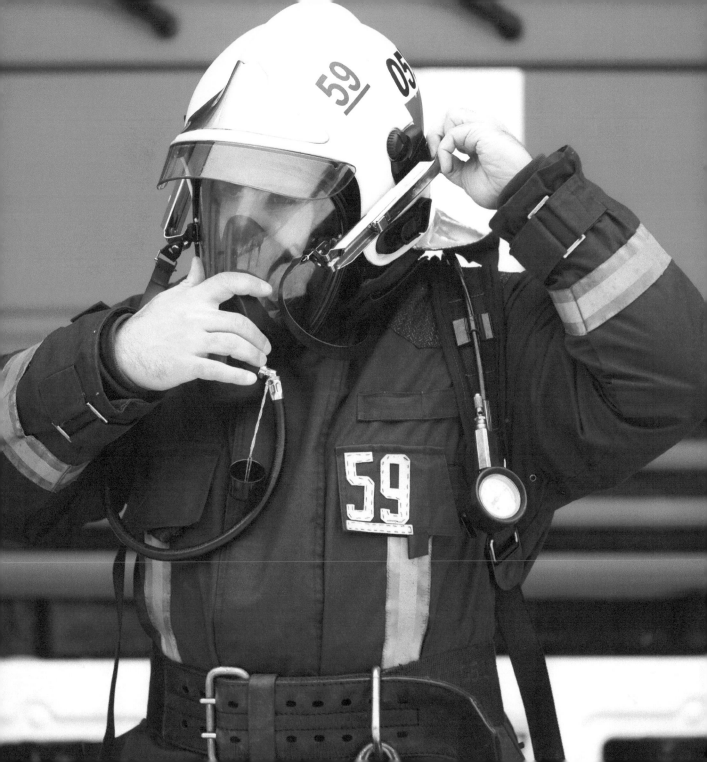

Scientists Wear Masks

Scientists explore how things work, make discoveries and solve problems. There are many different types of scientists.

They wear masks to protect their faces and lungs during science experiments.

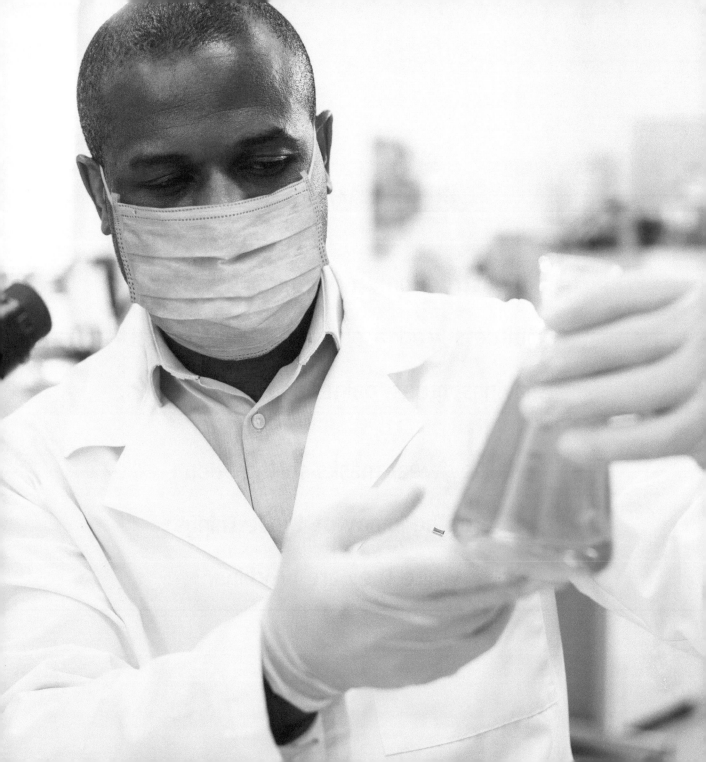

Builders Wear Masks

Construction workers, painters and builders work around wood and metal shavings, glues, paints and other smells.

They wear masks so they don't breathe in any of those things while they are working.

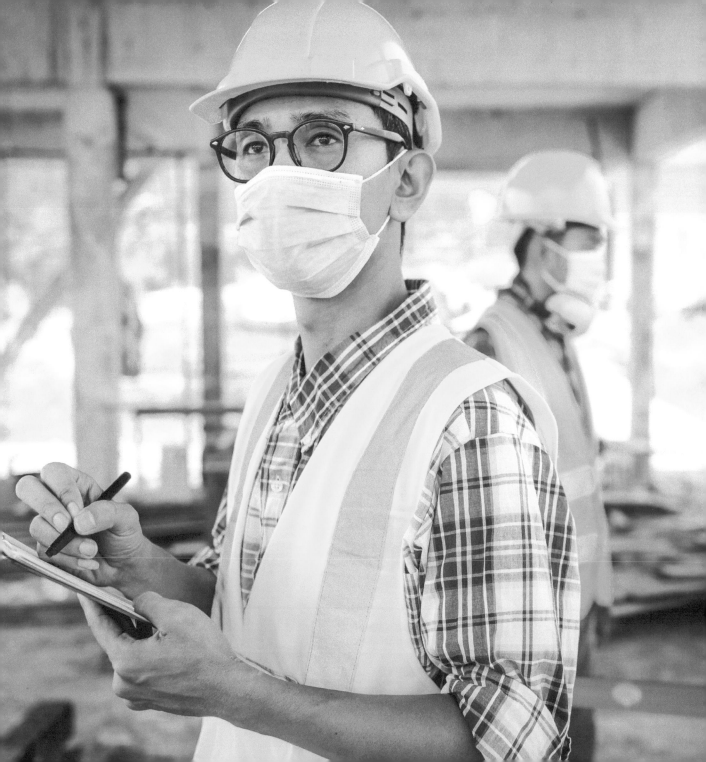

Doctors and Nurses Wear Masks

Many doctors and nurses help sick people.

When you are sick, you have yucky germs

that can make other people sick.

By wearing masks, doctors can keep

bad germs away and stay healthy.

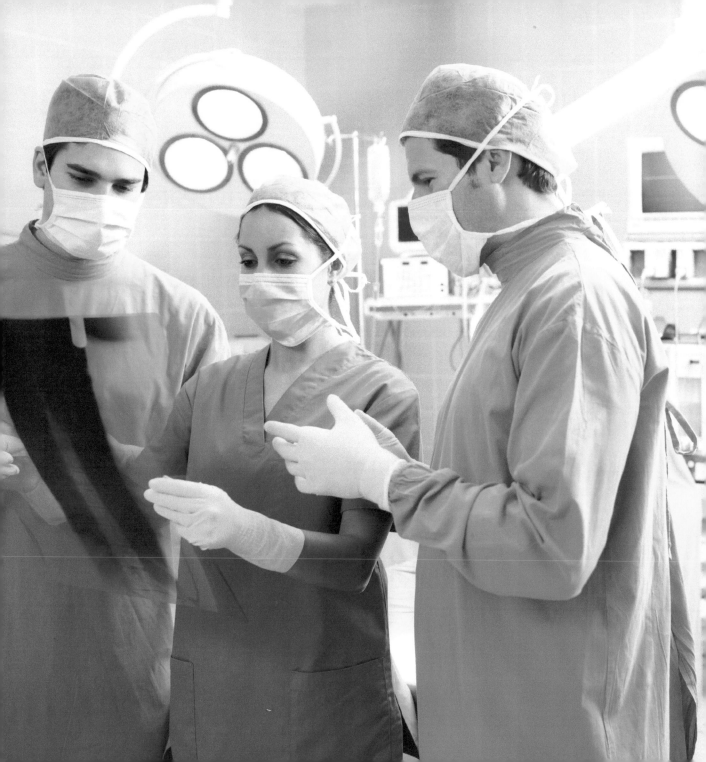

Veterinarians Wear Masks

Veterinarians take care of our pets just like doctors take care of us.

Like some doctors, Vets wear masks to keep from getting germs from animals and to keep from breathing in animal hairs or stinky smells!

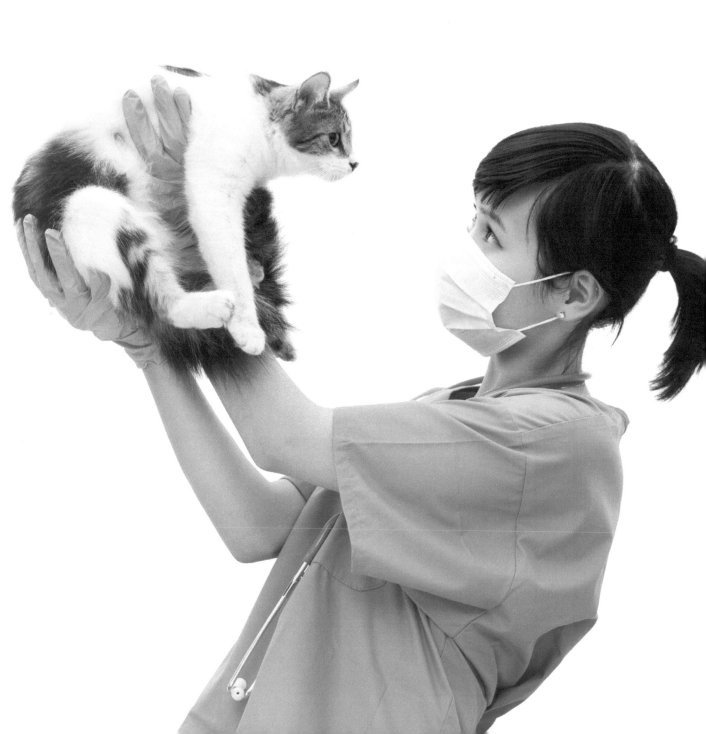

Landscapers Wear Masks

Landscapers, gardeners and mowers help trim grass, bushes and plants.

They wear masks to keep from breathing in dust, dirt and grass that might fly into their faces while they are working.

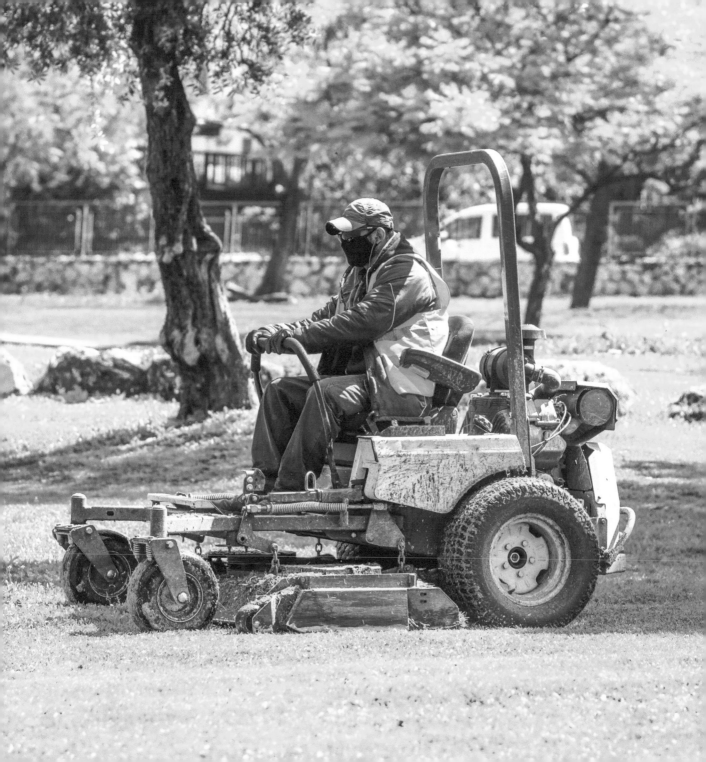

Athletes Wear Masks

Athletes, like football or hockey players, take a lot of bumps and falls while they are playing sports.

They wear masks and helmets to keep their heads and faces from getting hurt.

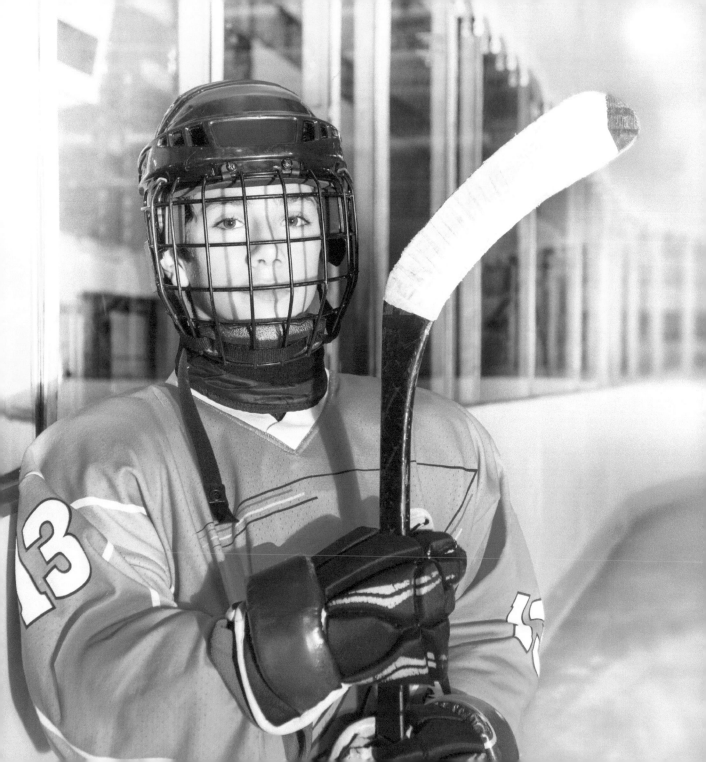

Astronauts Wear Masks

Astronauts are explorers and scientists who work in space.

People need air to breathe but there is no air in space. Astronauts wear special masks or helmets that hold in air for them to breathe.

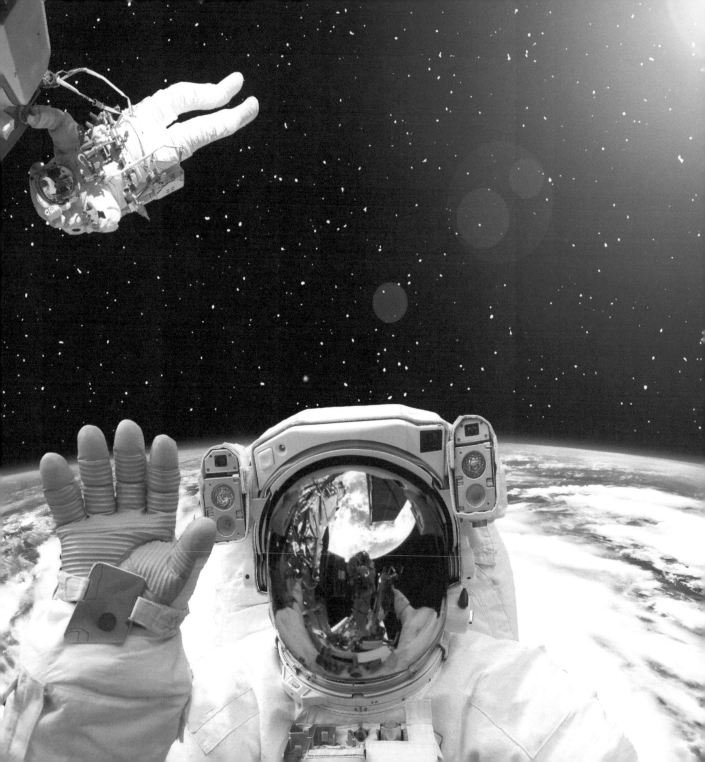

Scuba Divers Wear Masks

Snorkelers and scuba divers
explore life in the sea!

They wear masks to see and special
equipment to help them breathe
while they are underwater.

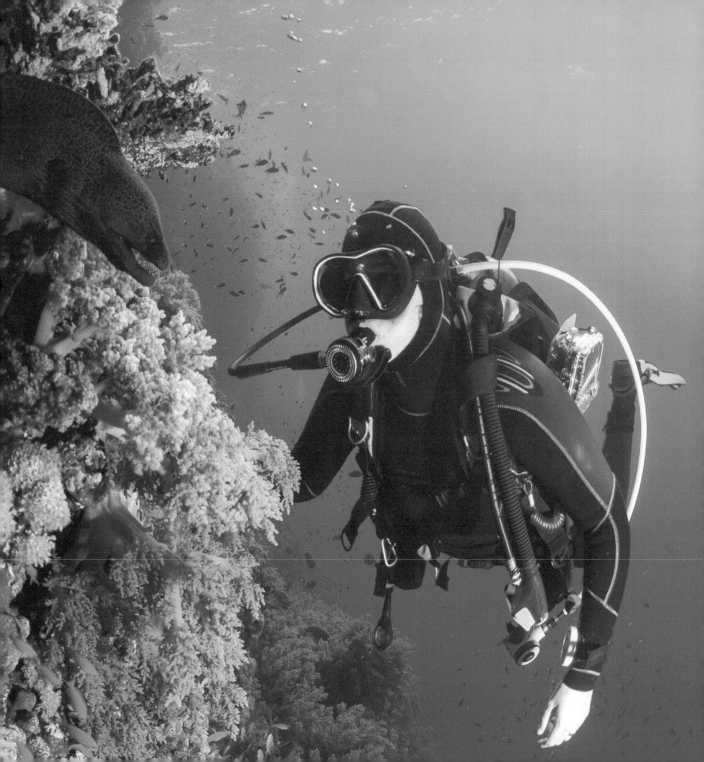

Beekeepers Wear Masks

Beekeepers are very brave.

They work around bees to get delicious honey.

Beekeepers wear masks

to protect their faces from bees

and especially from their stingers!

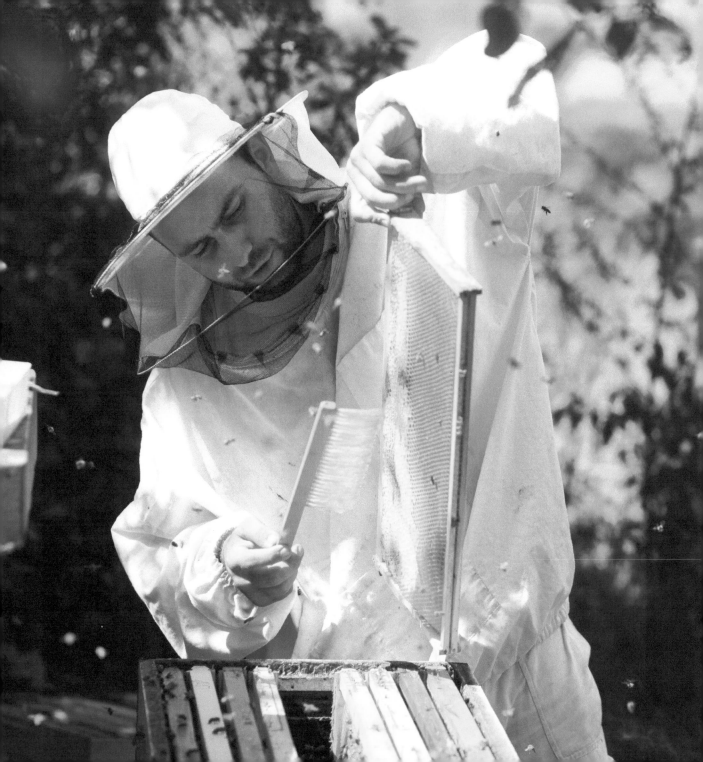

Skiers Wear Masks

Snow skiers go skiing down cold, icy and snowy mountains at very fast speeds.

They wear face masks to protect their faces from cold snow and air while they are speeding down the mountains! Brrr!

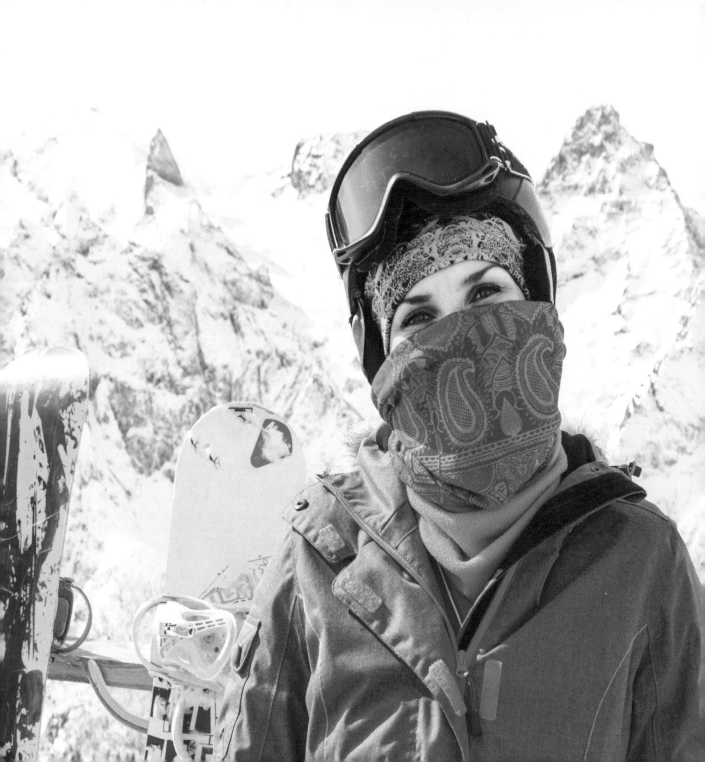

Superheroes Wear Masks

Superheroes are magical and mysterious!
They fight off bad guys and rescue people
while keeping their faces a secret!

Superheroes wear masks to
hide and protect their faces!

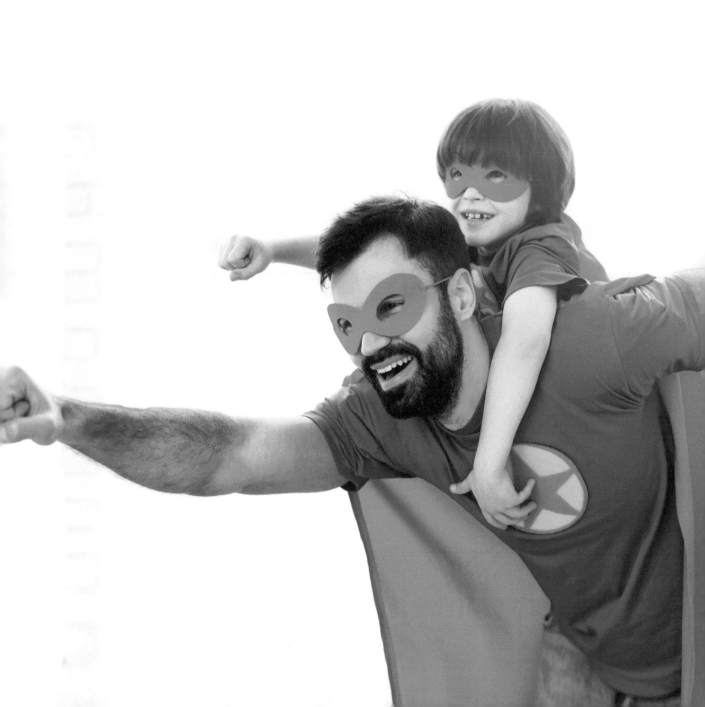

Grown-Ups Wear Masks

Mommies and daddies, aunts and uncles,

teachers and friends wear masks too.

Masks help to keep them from

spreading or getting germs

when they go out of the house.

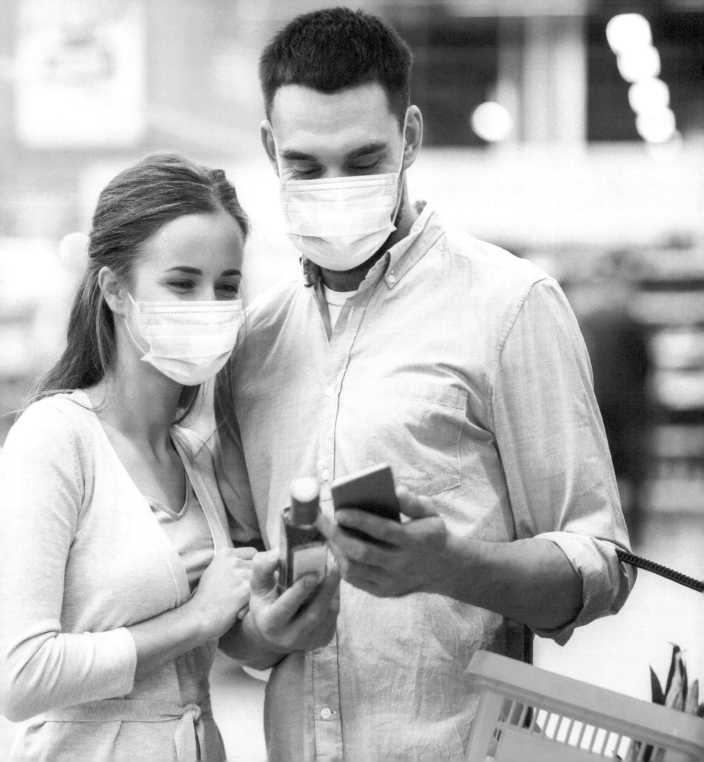

You Can Wear Masks

Just like grown-ups, when germs or viruses
are going around, you can wear masks too.

By wearing a mask, you can be the superhero
of your town and keep yourself and others safe.

A mask is only needed sometimes.
Don't worry – your parents will let you know
if and when you need to wear one.

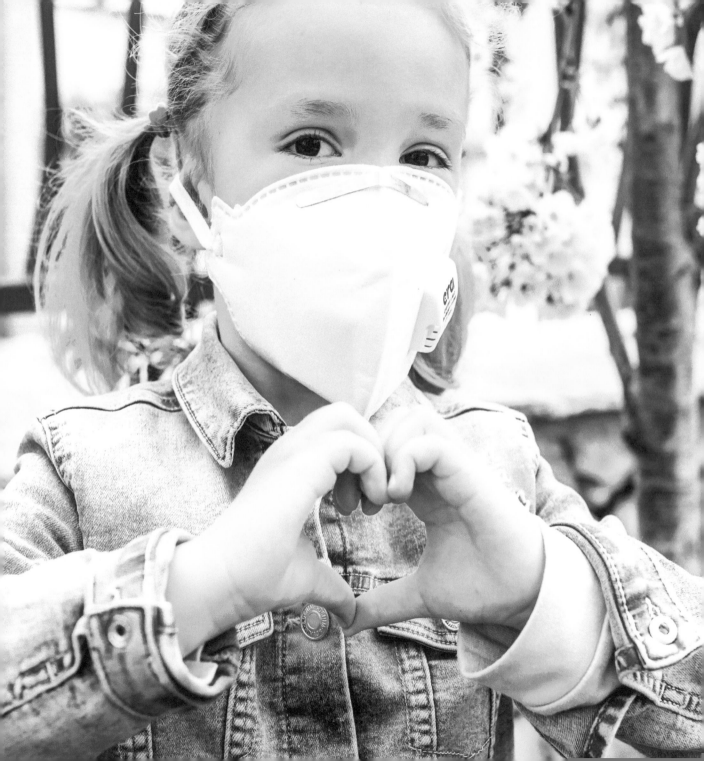

All About Masks

Masks might look a little funny,
but they are pretty awesome!

They protect people from many
different things, and they help
keep our community safe!

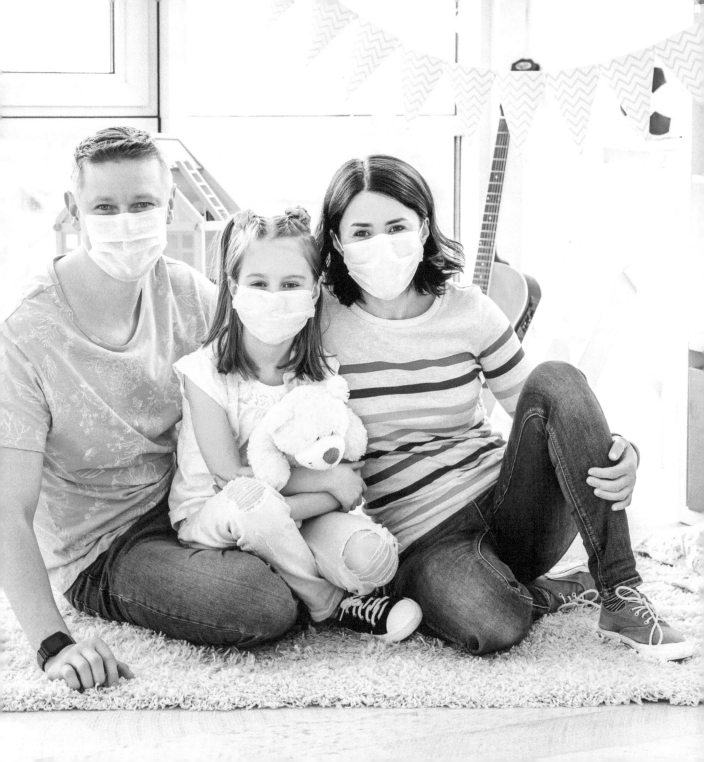

Now that you've learned all about masks,

you can ask your parent for your very own

superhero mask to take with you next time

you need to help save the day!

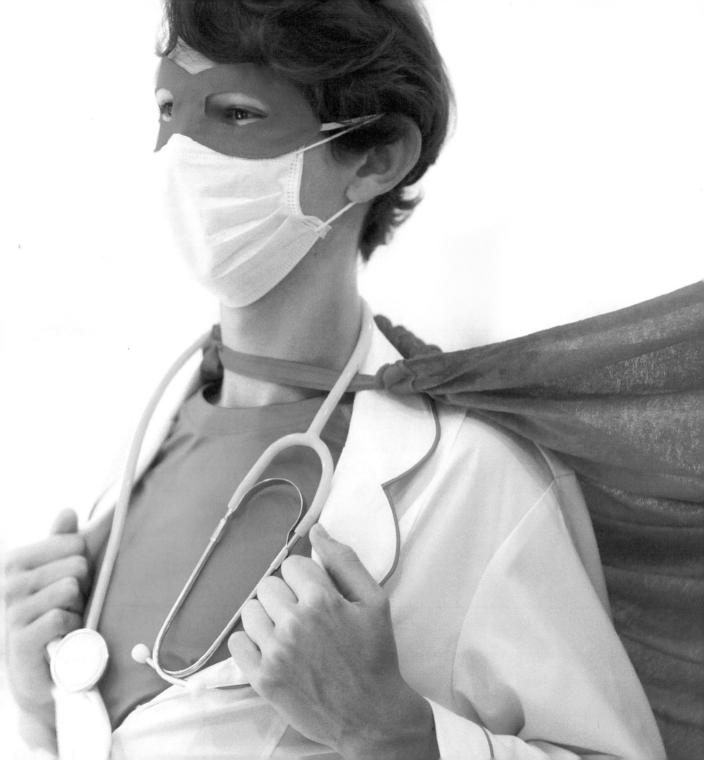

And don't forget - that
behind every mask...

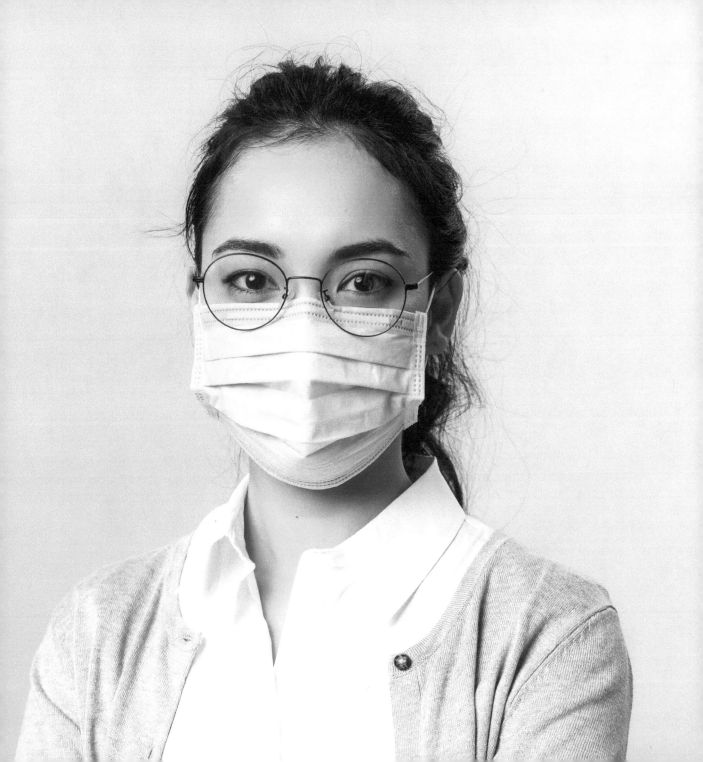

Is a friendly smile!

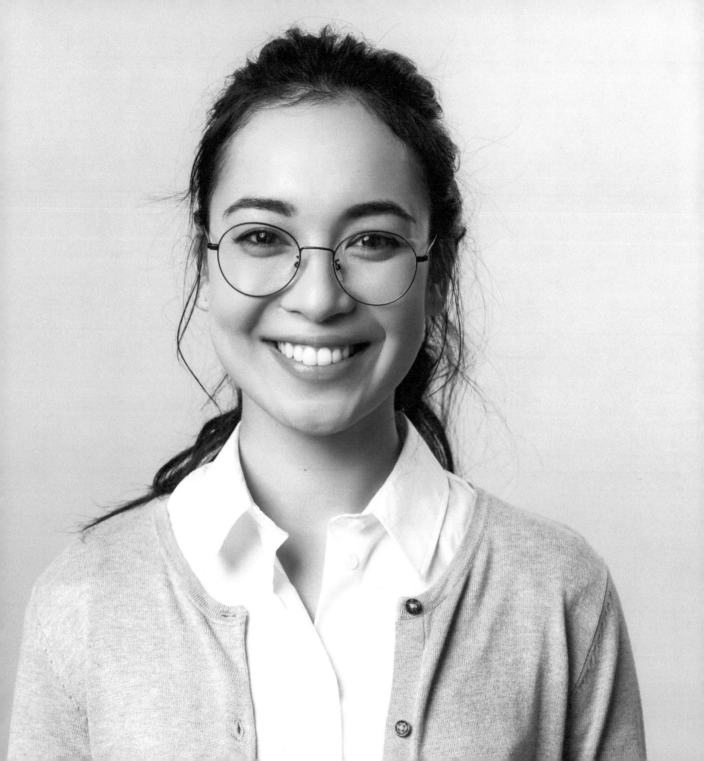

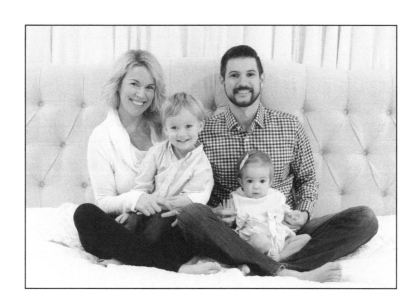

About the Author

Sara Jo Walker is a Nashville, Tennessee native, a public relations professional, a wife and a mother of two children. She works for a global media company doing media relations, event planning, communications and social media. Sara Jo is a graduate of the Mass Communications department at Middle Tennessee State University. She and her husband Ryan reside in Nashville with their two children, Jack and Ivy, and their cat Sake. This is her first book.

CPSIA information can be obtained
at www.ICGtesting.com
Printed in the USA
LVHW070228030820
662230LV00011B/935